Charles Lovjoy

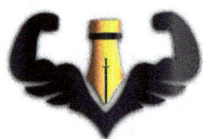

MUSCLE GANG PUBLICATIONS

# HEALTH IS WEALTH:

# HOLISTIC HOME REMEDIES

## By
## Charles Lovjoy

*Health Is Wealth: Holistic Home Remedies*

*Charles Lovjoy*

# HEALTH IS WEALTH: HOLISTIC HOME REMEDIES

**Copyright © 2024 Charles Lovjoy**

**FIRST EDITION ISBN:
978-1-7373302-6-4**

**Published by**

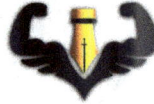

**MUSCLE GANG PUBLICATIONS**

**In association with**

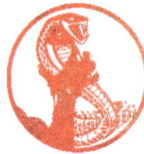

**TIC MADE ENTERTAINMENT**

## *Table of Contents:*

**Dedication**

**Disclaimer**

**Introduction**

**Chapter 1: The Transformative Power of Fasting** ..................................................................*1*

**Chapter 2: The Marvels of Sea Moss**..................*9*

**Chapter 3: God's Pharmacy: The Power of Herbs**...................................................*19*

**Chapter 4: Tackling Heartburn Naturally**............*27*

**Chapter 5: Herbs and Remedies to Eliminate Gas**.................................................*33*

**Chapter 6: Natural Remedies for Diarrhea**..........*39*

**Chapter 7: Natural Approaches to Managing Blood Pressure**..............................................*45*

**Chapter 8: Diabetes Management: Balancing Blood Sugar**..............................................*53*

## Table of Contents:

**Chapter 9: Health Benefits of Vinegar and Apple Cider Vinegar**............................................*63*

**Chapter 10: Health Benefits of Ginger**............................................*71*

**Chapter 11: The Multifaceted Benefits of Turmeric**............................................*79*

**Chapter 12: The Sweet Benefits of Cinnamon**............................................*87*

**Chapter 13: Natural Antibiotics**...............*93*

**Chapter 14: Embracing Holistic Habits for Optimal Health**............................................*99*

**Final Thoughts**.............................*105*

**Other Works**...........................................*109*

**References and Citations**.......................*113*

*Health Is Wealth: Holistic Home Remedies*

Charles Lovjoy

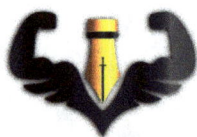

MUSCLE GANG PUBLICATIONS

## DEDICATION:

This book is dedicated to all the victims of the evil greedy pharmaceutical companies that caused the opioid epidemic. To everyone who has been told by doctors that they have to take medications with harmful side effects for the rest of their lives, I wrote this for you! My grandmother Alberta Simpson fell victim to complications from unnecessary prescription medications, so of course this is for her as well. I feel as though if I knew then what I know now, I could have saved my grandmother's life. Even though I can't bring my grandmother back, hopefully, this book will help save lives.

To my cousin Rhonda English, who was also a victim of the opioid crisis, till we meet again, I will dedicate my life to educating my people about the benefits of natural remedies and holistic healing.

To my uncles Kelvin Jerome Simpson and Henry Renard Simpson, I will do my best to protect the family just like you guys did before the untimely demise. To my aunt Winnie, you made me realize that "this time tomorrow, today will be yesterday," so I'm going to make the best of it right now. I love you all, Rest in peace.

To anyone suffering from preventable ailments and disease, and feels there is no hope, I'm here to let you know that the devil is a lie! There is hope! You don't have to be filthy rich to live a comfortable healthy life, and you can do so on your terms; just know that it's all about balance. I hope this book inspires each one to teach one. I wish you all health, wealth, and prosperity.

Health Is Wealth: Holistic Home Remedies

Charles Lovjoy

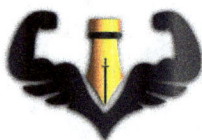

MUSCLE GANG PUBLICATIONS

## *Disclaimer*

The information provided in the book "Health Is Wealth," is intended for general informational purposes only and is not a substitute for professional medical advice, diagnosis, or treatment. The content within this book is based on research, holistic practices, nutritional insights, and scientific facts, but individual health conditions may vary. The information in this book is not intended to be a substitute for professional medical advice, diagnosis, or treatment. Always seek the advice of your physician or another qualified health provider with any questions you may have regarding a medical condition.

Each person is unique, and what works for one individual may not be suitable for another. It is crucial to consider individual health conditions, allergies, and sensitivities when exploring the recommendations provided.

This book discusses natural remedies and supplements, which may have potential benefits. However, it is important to consult with a healthcare professional before incorporating new remedies or supplements, especially if you are pregnant, nursing, taking medications, or have pre-existing health conditions.

Holistic living encompasses a broad range of practices that involve physical, mental, and spiritual aspects of well-being. It is recommended to integrate holistic practices mindfully and seek guidance if needed. Medical knowledge and holistic practices are continually evolving. The information in this book is current as of the knowledge cutoff date, and updates may occur. It is advisable to stay informed about developments in the field. The author and publisher disclaim any liability for any adverse effects or consequences resulting from the use or application of the information contained in this book.

*Health Is Wealth: Holistic Home Remedies*

Charles Lovjoy

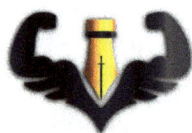

**MUSCLE GANG PUBLICATIONS**

# *Introduction:*

In the broad landscape of modern wellness, where pills and prescriptions often dominate humanity, "Health is Wealth: Holistic Home Remedies" emerges as a beacon of simplicity and wisdom. In our quest for better health, it's easy to overlook the cures that God has already provided. We must never forget the incredible healing power of nature, the very source from which life springs. This book is an invitation to rediscover that source.

Welcome to "Health Is Wealth: Holistic Home Remedies." In this comprehensive self-help guide, we embark on a journey to discover the incredible healing powers contained within the realms of natural herbs and substances. As we dive into each chapter, we'll explore practical remedies for common ailments such as heartburn, gas, diarrhea, high blood pressure, etcetera.

My mission is to empower you with knowledge, offering a holistic approach to wellness that is not only effective but also backed up by scientific facts that pharmaceutical companies don't want you to know. This book is more than just a collection of remedies; it's a roadmap to a healthier and more vibrant life.

As we embark on this journey, let's redefine the way we perceive healing. Natural remedies have been an integral part of human existence for centuries, rooted in the profound connection between humanity and the environment. In "Health Is Wealth," we rekindle this ancient bond, recognizing that true well-being is a harmonious interplay between mind, body, and nature.

The complexity of our health often feels like an intricate puzzle that is impossible for the average person to comprehend.

In this book, I simplify the pieces, providing a clear accessible guide to addressing common ailments. My approach is holistic, understanding that each chapter is a stepping stone towards a healthier, more balanced life. I invite you to explore the chapters not as standalone remedies but as interconnected facets of a comprehensive well-being strategy.

Knowledge is the key to empowerment. In "Health Is Wealth," I aim to empower you with insights into the healing potential of herbs and substances that may already be available in your home. Whether you're grappling with heartburn, gas, diarrhea, high blood pressure, or diabetes, this book offers practical solutions rooted in the richness of nature. It's an empowering journey towards taking charge of your health in a way that is both effective and sustainable.

While the subject matter of this book delves into the depths of holistic health, my commitment to readability remains unwavering. I understand the importance of making this information accessible to everyone, from seasoned health enthusiasts to curious 7th-grade readers. The language is crafted with clarity, ensuring that the wisdom shared resonates with all, fostering a community of empowered individuals on a shared path to well-being.

"Health is Wealth" is more than a guide; it's an affirmation of the transformative power within you. Each chapter unfolds as a revelation, unraveling the secrets of natural remedies and inviting you to embrace a lifestyle that celebrates the simplicity and potency of nature. This book is a testament to the belief that healing is not controlled by government institutions and pharmaceutical companies but a continuous, enriching journey controlled by the people.

Understanding the principles behind holistic health sets the stage for the transformative journey that follows. We will discuss the relationship between nature and our well-being, emphasizing the importance of embracing natural remedies in our daily lives. With all that said, let us dive into the historical roots of natural healing practices, unveiling the wisdom passed down through generations. By the end of this book, you'll be equipped with the knowledge needed to embark on your personal healing journey, harnessing the power of nature to enhance your overall health.

# Chapter 1: The Transformative Power Of Fasting

I do not believe in saving the best for last; I'm going to give you the best right now! In this chapter, we will explore the profound benefits of my favorite holistic remedy, fasting. Fasting is a practice that extends beyond the mere absence of food to become a transformative journey for the body and mind. From cellular regeneration to enhanced mental clarity, I believe fasting is the most effective remedy of all.

If you think about it, what's the first thing doctors tell you to do before coming in for an appointment? That's right, they tell you to fast from 6 to 12 hours before your visit. Fasting unveils a spectrum of advantages that span various durations, from a 24-hour fast to extended periods lasting up to 7 days.

## A. The Cellular Renewal Symphony

### 1. Autophagy Activation:

- Fasting triggers autophagy, a cellular cleaning process where the body disposes of damaged or weak cells. This renewal process contributes to overall cellular health and longevity.

### 2. Mitochondrial Enhancement:

- Fasting supports mitochondrial health, improving the efficiency of energy production within cells and promoting resilience against oxidative stress.

### 3. Stem Cell Activation:

- Extended fasts stimulate the production of new stem cells, fostering regeneration and repair throughout various tissues and organs.

## B. The Fasting Spectrum: Benefits Across Durations

### 1. 24-Hour Fast:

- Cellular Reset: A 24-hour fast initiates the process of autophagy, providing a quick cellular reset.
- Blood Sugar Regulation: Fasting for a day helps stabilize blood sugar levels.

### 2. 48-Hour Fast:

- Enhanced Autophagy: Extended fasting further intensifies autophagy, promoting deeper cellular cleansing.
- Mental Clarity: Some individuals report heightened mental clarity and focus during a 48-hour fast.

### 3. 72-Hour Fast:

- Optimized Insulin Sensitivity: A 72-hour fast contributes to improved insulin sensitivity, potentially reducing the risk of type 2 diabetes.

- Gut Rest: Fasting allows the digestive system to rest, promoting gut health.

### 4. 5-Day Fast:

- Deep Cellular Regeneration: A longer fast enhances the process of stem cell activation, promoting profound cellular regeneration.
- Immune System Rejuvenation: Fasting supports immune function by clearing out old immune cells and generating new, healthier ones.

### 5. 7-Day Fast:

- Metabolic Reset: A week-long fast may contribute to a metabolic reset, promoting better weight management.
- Emotional Detox: Extended fasting can provide emotional clarity and a reset in the relationship with food.

## C. Nourishing the Body During Fasting

### 1. Hydration:

- Water: Stay well-hydrated with plain water to support bodily functions and aid in the elimination of toxins.

### 2. Electrolytes:

- Coconut Water: Rich in electrolytes, coconut water helps maintain hydration and supports mineral balance.
- Broth: Bone broth provides essential minerals and electrolytes, contributing to overall well-being.

### 3. Tea and Coffee:

- Herbal Teas: Caffeine-free herbal teas offer a soothing and hydrating option during fasting.
- Black Coffee: A cup of black coffee can provide a gentle energy boost and may enhance mental alertness.

### 4. Supplements:

- Multivitamins: Consider taking a multivitamin to ensure essential nutrient intake.
- Electrolyte Supplements: Especially crucial for longer fasts to prevent electrolyte imbalances.

**5. Breaking the Fast:**

- Gentle Foods: When reintroducing food, start with easily digestible, nutrient-dense options like fruits or vegetables.
- Probiotics: Incorporate probiotic-rich foods to support gut health as you resume regular eating.

## D. The Mind-Body Connection

### 1. Enhanced Mental Clarity:

- Fasting has been linked to increased focus, mental clarity, and a sense of heightened awareness.

## 2. Emotional Resilience:

- The discipline of fasting can cultivate emotional resilience, offering a mindful approach to eating and fostering a healthier relationship with food.

When done consistently, fasting is a natural way for your body to reset and recharge itself. Here's a fun fact: the average adult human has enough fat and nutrients stored in the body to survive 21 to 40 days before the body enters a state of starvation. Hydration plays a crucial role in survival. While a person may survive without food for weeks, the absence of water can lead to dehydration much more quickly. The duration one can survive without water varies based on factors such as climate, physical activity, and individual health.

Embarking on a fasting journey requires thoughtful consideration and attention to your body's signals. Whether you choose a shorter intermittent fast or explore extended fasting, it's essential to listen to your body and seek guidance if needed. Fasting is a personal experience, and its benefits can vary among individuals.

Fasting, especially extended fasting, should be approached with caution and under the guidance of a healthcare professional. Individuals with certain medical conditions or those taking medications may require tailored advice.

## Chapter 2: The Marvels Of Sea Moss

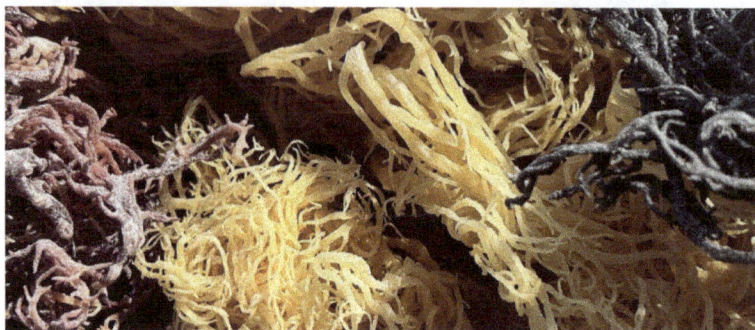

Embark on a journey into the depths of the ocean with Chapter 2 of "Health Is Wealth," where we unravel the mysteries of sea moss—a potent marine marvel celebrated for its rich nutrient profile and supreme health benefits. From essential vitamins and minerals to its potential role in addressing various ailments, sea moss emerges as a powerhouse of natural wellness and is also my second favorite remedy next to fasting. The reason sea moss gel is my second favorite natural remedy is that you can consume it while fasting to ensure that the body will not go into nutrient or vitamin deficiency.

I have a personal testimony about sea moss. At the time of writing this book, I am a 45-year-old man. From around the age of 25 to 40 years old, I used to get terrible sinus infections at least once every other month until I stumbled across a mini-documentary about the benefits of sea moss.

I found the documentary to be very intriguing, so I tried it. To my surprise, I haven't had a sinus infection since the day I introduced sea moss into my life. Enough about me, let's dive into the wonderful marvels of sea moss.

## A. The Nutrient Bounty of Sea Moss

### 1. Vitamins:

- Vitamin A: Essential for vision, immune function, and skin health.
- Vitamin B2 (Riboflavin): Supports energy production and red blood cell formation.
- Vitamin B9 (Folate): Crucial for DNA synthesis and cell division.
- Vitamin C: Boosts immune function and promotes collagen formation.
- Vitamin E: An antioxidant that protects cells from oxidative stress.

### 2. Minerals:

- Iodine: Vital for thyroid function and hormone production.
- Iron: Essential for oxygen transport in the blood.
- Zinc: Supports immune function and wound healing.
- Calcium: Crucial for bone health and muscle function.
- Magnesium: Aids in muscle and nerve function, energy production, and bone health.
- Phosphorus: Important for bone and teeth formation.

**3. Fiber:**

- Sea moss provides a significant amount of dietary fiber, promoting digestive health and supporting a feeling of fullness.

**4. Antioxidants:**

- Antioxidants in sea moss help neutralize free radicals, protecting cells from damage.

**5. Essential Fatty Acids:**

- Sea moss contains omega-3 and omega-6 fatty acids, supporting heart health and overall well-being.

**B. Health Benefits of Sea Moss**

**1. Thyroid Support:**

- Iodine content in sea moss contributes to thyroid health, potentially aiding in the regulation of metabolism.

**2. Immune Boost:**

- Vitamins A and C, along with antioxidants, bolster the immune system, enhancing the body's ability to fight infections.

**3. Gut Health:**

- The rich fiber content supports digestive health by promoting regular bowel movements and fostering a healthy gut microbiome.

**4. Joint and Bone Support:**

- Calcium, magnesium, and phosphorus in sea moss contribute to bone health, potentially reducing the risk of osteoporosis.

**5. Skin Radiance:**

- Vitamins A, E, and C, combined with antioxidants, promote skin health, potentially reducing signs of aging.

**6. Energy Boost:**

- Sea moss's iron content supports oxygen transport, combating fatigue and promoting overall energy levels.

**7. Cardiovascular Health:**

   Omega-3 fatty acids contribute to heart health by reducing inflammation and supporting optimal cardiovascular function.

**8. Blood Sugar Regulation:**

- Sea moss may play a role in managing blood sugar levels, making it a potential ally for those with diabetes.

### C. Addressing Ailments with Sea Moss

**1. Respiratory Issues:**

- Sea moss's mucilaginous properties may help soothe respiratory issues, making it beneficial for conditions like bronchitis.

## 2. Digestive Disorders:

- The fiber in sea moss supports digestive health, potentially alleviating symptoms of conditions like irritable bowel syndrome (IBS).

## 3. Joint Pain and Inflammation:

- Sea moss's anti-inflammatory properties may offer relief for joint pain and inflammation associated with conditions like arthritis.

## 4. Thyroid Disorders:

- Iodine content in sea moss may support thyroid function, potentially aiding in the management of thyroid disorders.

### D. Incorporating Sea Moss into Your Routine

## 1. Smoothies:

- Blend sea moss into your favorite smoothies for a nutrient-packed boost.

## 2. Soups and Stews:

- Add sea moss to soups and stews for nutritional enhancement and a subtle thickening effect.

## 3. Beverages:

- Prepare sea moss-infused beverages or teas for a refreshing way to reap its benefits.

Sea moss can be consumed in many forms: whole plant form, powder, capsules, or gel; all of which can be purchased at your local health food store. However, my personal preference is in gel form. In order to make sea moss gel, you will need to do the following:

1. Place sea moss in a large container, soak the sea moss plant in purified or alkaline water for a half hour.

2. Rinse and repeat to ensure removal of debris

3. Add 2 capfuls of lemon or lime juice and enough purified water to cover the sea moss.

4. Refrigerate for 24 hours.

5. Place the contents of the container into a blender and blend for 1 minute for proper gel-like consistency.

6. Now you can add the fruit of your choice and blend for another minute.

It's important to note that sea moss can be frozen for up to 6 months and refrigerated for up to 1 month before going bad. While sea moss offers numerous health benefits, moderation is key. Excessive consumption may lead to an imbalance in certain nutrients and dehydration. About 1 to 2 tablespoons per day is all that is needed. Consult with healthcare professionals before embarking on this journey, especially if you have pre-existing health conditions or are taking medications. Sea moss may aggravate any fish or shellfish allergies.

## <u>*Chapter 3: God's Pharmacy: The Power of Herbs*</u>

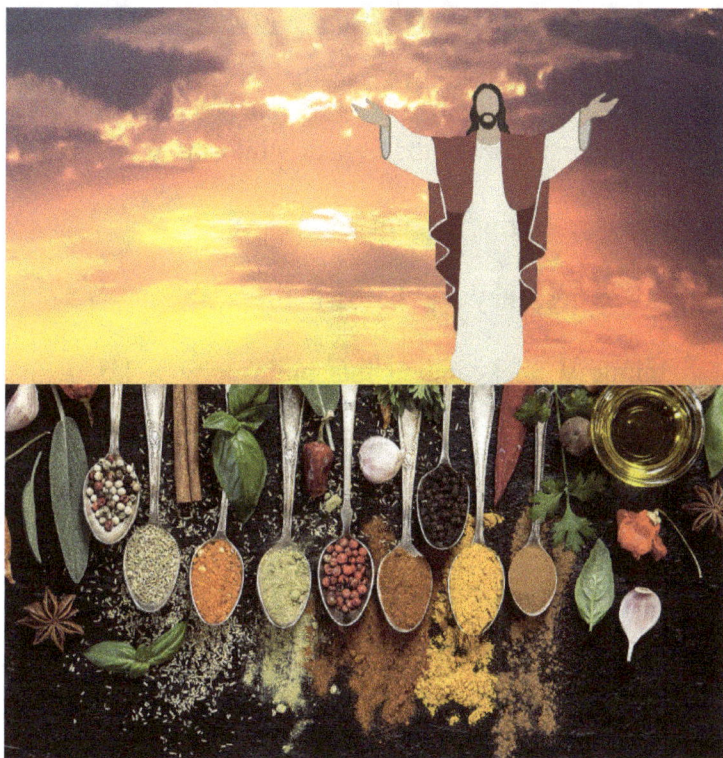

Join us on a captivating journey into the heart of what I like to call God's pharmacy, where the vibrant hues and fragrances of herbs weave a tapestry of healing. Chapter 3 of "Health is Wealth" is a portal into the profound world of herbal remedies—a realm where ancient wisdom meets contemporary well-being.

**17**

## 1. *The Holistic Philosophy of Herbal Healing*

Before we dive into the specifics of individual herbs, let us first discuss the holistic philosophy concerning herbal healing. Herbs are not merely substances with medicinal properties; they are the basis for which all medicines try to mimic. Understanding this philosophy is key to unlocking the full potential of herbs in promoting holistic health.

Herbs, with their diverse array of bioactive compounds, offer a holistic approach to wellness. From antioxidants that combat oxidative stress to anti-inflammatory agents that soothe bodily discomfort, each herb contributes a unique therapeutic element. "The Power of Herbs" aims to demystify this intricate dance of compounds, making it accessible to readers of all backgrounds.

## 2. *Exploring the Herbaceous Symphony*

Our exploration takes us through a botanical symphony where each herb plays a distinct note. Chamomile, with its delicate flowers, becomes a soothing melody for stress and insomnia. Lavender, with its aromatic blooms, emerges as a calming harmony, easing anxiety and promoting restful sleep. Peppermint, with its invigorating essence, transforms into a refreshing tune for digestive woes.

We delve into the stories behind these herbs, weaving narratives that span cultures and centuries. The ancient Egyptians valued chamomile for its healing properties, using it in teas and salves for its calming effects. Lavender found its place in the medieval gardens of Europe, where it was employed not only for its fragrance but also for its antiseptic properties. Peppermint, with its versatile uses, has roots in ancient traditions across Asia and the Middle East, where it was embraced for its digestive benefits.

**19**

## 3. *Cultural Wisdom of Herbal Healing*

Throughout history, diverse cultures have harnessed the healing power of herbs, leaving behind a rich patchwork of traditional wisdom. In traditional Chinese medicine, ginseng has been revered for centuries as an adaptogen, believed to restore and invigorate the body's balance. Ayurveda, the ancient healing system of India, celebrates the holistic properties of turmeric, using it for its anti-inflammatory and antioxidant effects.

In Native American traditions, echinacea was valued for its immune-boosting properties, while in South America, the healing traditions of the Amazon rainforest introduced the world to the wonders of plants like cat's claw. Each culture, with its unique environment and traditions, has contributed to the global reservoir of herbal knowledge, showcasing the universality of relying on nature for healing.

## 4. The Rich History of Chinese Herbalism

China, with its ancient civilization, has a profound history of herbal medicine. Traditional Chinese medicine (TCM) is a holistic system that views the body as an interconnected network, and herbs play a pivotal role in restoring balance. Ginseng, known as "Ren Shen," is a cornerstone of Chinese herbalism. Believed to boost energy, promote longevity, and strengthen the body's vital forces, ginseng has been cherished for its adaptogenic properties.

Another revered herb in Chinese herbalism is Astragalus, known as "Huang Qi." Used for centuries, Astragalus is considered an immune system tonic, supporting overall vitality. The Chinese herbal tradition emphasizes the importance of balance and harmony, and many herbal formulas are designed to address the root causes of ailments rather than merely alleviating symptoms.

21

## 5. *Ayurveda: the Symphony of Spices*

Ayurveda, the ancient healing system of India, is a holistic approach that recognizes individual constitution and seeks to bring balance to the body, mind, and spirit. Turmeric, known as "Haldi" in Sanskrit, is a golden-hued spice celebrated for its anti-inflammatory and antioxidant properties. Ayurvedic practitioners use turmeric to support joint health, aid digestion, and promote overall well-being.

The Ayurvedic tradition also incorporates a symphony of spices, each with its unique contribution to health. Cinnamon, cardamom, ginger, and cloves are often used in Ayurvedic formulations for their warming and digestive properties. The holistic approach of Ayurveda extends beyond the physical, addressing emotional and spiritual well-being through the use of herbs and lifestyle practices.

## 6. *Native American Traditions*

Indigenous cultures in North America have a deep connection with the land and its healing gifts. Echinacea, also known as the purple coneflower, holds a special place in Native American herbalism. Used by Plains Indian tribes, echinacea was traditionally employed to support the immune system and aid in recovery from various ailments.

The Native American healing approach often involves a holistic perspective, viewing health as a harmonious balance between the individual and the surrounding environment. Herbal remedies are integrated into ceremonial practices, creating a healing circle that encompasses physical, spiritual, and communal well-being.

## 7. *Amazon Rainforest: Cat's Claw and the Wisdom of the Jungle*

In the heart of the Amazon rainforest, indigenous communities have long relied on the rich biodiversity of the jungle for their health and sustenance. Cat's Claw, known as "Una de Gato," is a woody vine revered for its immune-boosting properties.

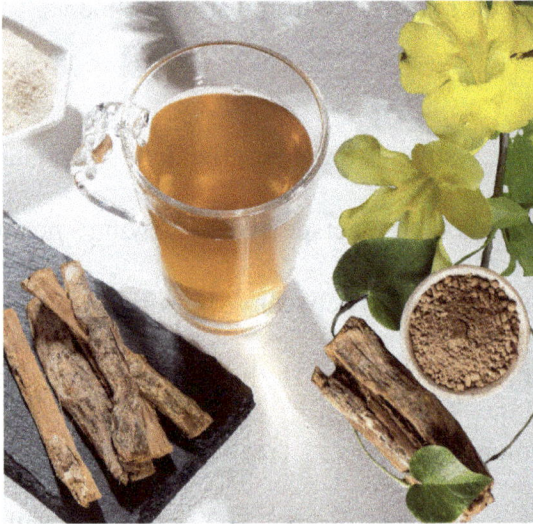

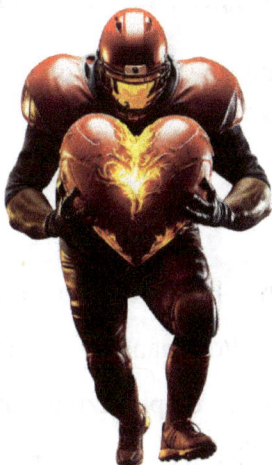

## *Chapter 4: Heartburn* — *Tackling Naturally*

This chapter will guide you in crafting your personalized heartburn toolkit, incorporating herbal remedies, dietary considerations, and lifestyle adjustments. By the end, you'll have a comprehensive understanding of how to navigate and mitigate heartburn symptoms naturally, fostering a sense of empowerment over your digestive well-being.

Before we dive into the subject of heartburn and its remedies, let us gain insight into the nature of heartburn. Often caused by stomach acid flowing back into the esophagus, heartburn can lead to a burning sensation in the chest.

Understanding the triggers, such as certain foods, stress, or lifestyle habits, forms the foundation for crafting effective and sustainable solutions.

Besides herbs, lifestyle adjustments play a crucial role in preventing and/or managing heartburn. We explore dietary modifications, emphasizing the importance of mindful eating and identifying trigger foods. Practical tips for stress management and maintaining a healthy weight are also integral components of our holistic approach. As we dive deeper into the realm of natural remedies, let us discuss a few herbal allies in the war against heartburn.

1. **Peppermint**: Known for its soothing properties, peppermint aids in relaxing the muscles of the gastrointestinal tract. This not only helps in reducing discomfort but also supports smoother digestion, especially when used as a tea.
2. **Fennel**: With its gentle, aromatic flavor, fennel has been used traditionally to ease digestive issues.
   Fennel seeds can be chewed after meals to promote digestion and alleviate heartburn symptoms. They possess carminative properties, helping to reduce gas and bloating.

3. **Aloe Vera:** Beyond its topical applications, aloe vera offers internal benefits for digestive health. Drinking aloe vera juice may help soothe irritation in the esophagus and stomach lining. It's crucial to choose aloe vera products specifically intended for internal use and consult with a healthcare professional before incorporating them into your routine.

4. **DGL Licorice:** Deglycyrrhizinated licorice, or DGL, is a modified form of licorice root that retains its digestive benefits without the side effects.

   DGL licorice can help soothe and protect the mucous lining of the stomach and esophagus.

5. **Turmeric:** Widely recognized for its anti-inflammatory properties, turmeric can play a role in alleviating heartburn symptoms. Curcumin, the active compound in turmeric, may help reduce inflammation in the digestive tract. Incorporating turmeric into your diet or taking it as a supplement can contribute to overall digestive wellness.

6. **Chamomile Tea:** Chamomile tea has anti-inflammatory properties and may help calm the digestive tract. Sip on chamomile tea after meals.

7. **Baking Soda:** Mix a teaspoon of baking soda in a glass of water and drink it slowly. Baking soda can help neutralize stomach acid, but use it sparingly.

8. **Ginger**: Fresh ginger, whether in tea or as a supplement, may help reduce heartburn symptoms due to its anti-inflammatory properties.

9. **Slippery Elm**: available in supplement or tea form, can coat and soothe the digestive tract, potentially easing heartburn.

10. **Papaya Enzymes**: Papaya contains enzymes, such as papain, which aid in digestion. Chewable papaya enzyme tablets may help prevent heartburn.

## *Chapter 5: Herbs and Remedies to Eliminate Gas*

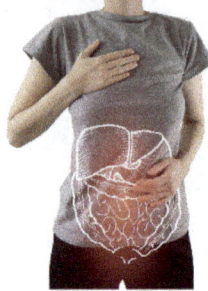

As we dive further into the intricacies of digestive well-being, this chapter expands its focus to explore additional herbs and remedies specifically aimed at eliminating gas and promoting a more comfortable digestive experience. On the road to digestive harmony, here are a few herbs that will help eliminate gas:

1. **Fennel Seeds:** Chewed after meals, fennel seeds act as a natural carminative, helping to relieve gas and bloating. Fennel tea is another delightful way to incorporate this herb into your routine.Fennel seeds not only provide a pleasant, licorice-like flavor but also offer significant relief from gas and bloating.

The volatile oils in fennel seeds help relax the muscles of the gastrointestinal tract, reducing spasms that contribute to gas. Chew a teaspoon of fennel seeds after meals or brew a soothing cup of fennel tea for digestive comfort.

2. **Caraway Seeds:** Known for their carminative and antimicrobial properties, caraway seeds aid in digestion and reduce gas. Consuming caraway seeds or using them in cooking can be beneficial for alleviating digestive discomfort.

3. **Anise:** With its sweet, licorice-like flavor, anise has carminative properties that can help reduce gas and soothe the digestive tract. Anise tea or incorporating crushed anise seeds into dishes adds a flavorful touch.

4. **Cumin:** Renowned for its digestive benefits, cumin can help prevent gas and bloating. Including cumin in your cooking or sipping on cumin tea can aid in promoting digestive comfort. Cumin, a staple in many spice cabinets, is celebrated for its digestive properties. It stimulates the secretion of digestive enzymes, aiding in the breakdown of food and reducing the likelihood of gas formation. Incorporate ground cumin into your cooking, or brew a cup of cumin tea to support digestive well-being.

5. **Activated Charcoal:** While not an herb, activated charcoal is a natural remedy that can absorb excess gas in the digestive system. Taken in supplement form, it may help alleviate bloating and discomfort caused by gas.

Everyone's body has different triggers, so it is very important to listen and pay close attention to your body. In addition to the herbs and remedies previously mentioned, holistic lifestyle practices also contribute to effective gas relief. Here are 3 helpful tips that may help reduce gas:

1. **Mindful Eating**

Practice mindful eating to enhance digestion. Chew your food thoroughly, savor each bite, and eat in a relaxed environment. This mindful approach can help prevent overeating and reduce the likelihood of gas formation.

2. **Stay Hydrated**

Adequate hydration is crucial for maintaining a healthy digestive system. Drinking water throughout the day supports the smooth movement of food through the digestive tract, reducing the chances of gas accumulation.

3. **Physical Activity**

Incorporate regular physical activity into your routine. Exercise promotes overall digestive health by stimulating the muscles of the digestive tract, preventing stagnation and reducing the likelihood of gas-related discomfort.

This chapter concludes by emphasizing the importance of crafting a comprehensive digestive toolkit that addresses various aspects of digestive well-being. Whether you're targeting heartburn, gas, or overall digestive harmony, the combination of herbal allies, dietary considerations, and lifestyle practices forms a holistic approach to digestive health.

"Health Is Wealth" continues to unfold as a comprehensive guide, empowering you to embrace a lifestyle that nurtures your digestive system.

In the subsequent chapters, we will explore more facets of natural wellness, offering insights and practical tools for your journey to a healthier, balanced life.

Remember, individual responses to remedies may vary, and it's essential to consult with a healthcare professional, especially if heartburn is persistent or severe.

Lifestyle and dietary changes, along with natural remedies, can contribute to managing and preventing heartburn.

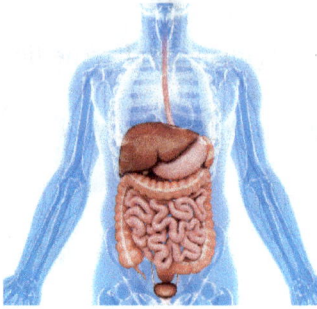

## *Chapter 6: Natural Remedies for Diarrhea*

In the intricate symphony of digestive health, occasional disruptions like diarrhea can disrupt the entire rhythm. Chapter 6 of "Health Is Wealth" takes a closer look at the natural herbs and remedies available to reclaim digestive balance when faced with diarrhea. Understanding the causes, implementing effective remedies, and embracing preventive measures form the core of this exploration.

Before delving into remedies, let us gain insights into the nature of diarrhea. Whether caused by viral infections, bacterial imbalances, or dietary indiscretions, diarrhea disrupts the normal absorption of water and nutrients in the intestines, leading to increased frequency and fluidity of bowel movements.

The impact of diarrhea extends beyond physical discomfort, affecting hydration levels, nutrient absorption, and overall well-being. Recognizing the underlying causes is crucial for tailoring effective and holistic solutions. Here are a few remedies and herbal allies in the war against diarrhea:

**1. Psyllium Husk:** Psyllium husk, a soluble fiber, can help bulk up stools and absorb excess water, providing relief from watery diarrhea. It also supports overall digestive health by promoting regular bowel movements.

**2. Banana:** Known for its binding properties, ripe bananas can help firm up loose stools. They are gentle on the stomach and provide essential nutrients, making them a valuable choice during bouts of diarrhea.

**3. Ginger:** Renowned for its anti-inflammatory and antimicrobial properties, ginger can help soothe the digestive tract. Ginger tea or adding fresh ginger to meals can aid in reducing inflammation and easing diarrhea symptoms.

**4. Activated Charcoal:** Activated charcoal, known for its ability to absorb toxins, can be effective in binding to substances causing diarrhea. It's crucial to use activated charcoal supplements as directed for short-term relief.

**5. Chamomile Tea:** Chamomile's anti-inflammatory and calming properties extend to the digestive system. Chamomile tea can help relax the intestinal muscles, alleviating cramps and discomfort associated with diarrhea.

**6. White Rice:** Plain white rice is a bland and easily digestible food that can help firm up stools. It's part of the BRAT diet (bananas, rice, applesauce, and toast) often recommended for diarrhea.

**7. Apple Sauce:** Unsweetened applesauce is gentle on the stomach and provides pectin, which may help bulk up stools.

**8. Blueberries:** Blueberries have antioxidant properties and may help alleviate diarrhea. They can be eaten by themselves, mixed in a smoothie, or added to yogurt.

**9. Coconut Water**: Coconut water is a natural source of electrolytes and can help prevent dehydration during diarrhea.

**10. Peppermint Tea**: Peppermint tea has anti-inflammatory and antispasmodic properties that may help soothe the digestive tract and alleviate diarrhea.

In a nutshell, here are the 4 most important things to remember when dealing with diarrhea:

**1. Hydration and Electrolyte Balance**

Diarrhea often leads to dehydration and electrolyte imbalances. Replenishing fluids and essential electrolytes is paramount for recovery. Consider oral rehydration solutions, coconut water, and clear broths to ensure adequate hydration.

**2. Dietary Considerations during Diarrhea**

Adjusting your diet during episodes of diarrhea is crucial for supporting digestive healing.

Opt for easily digestible foods such as rice, plain crackers, boiled potatoes, and cooked carrots. Avoid dairy, caffeine, and high-fiber foods temporarily.

### 3. Probiotics for Gut Restoration

Introducing probiotics can aid in restoring the balance of beneficial bacteria in the gut. Yogurt with live cultures, kefir, and fermented foods like sauerkraut can contribute to a healthier gut environment.

### 4. When to Seek Medical Attention

While natural remedies can provide relief for mild cases of diarrhea, it's essential to seek medical attention if:

- Diarrhea persists for more than a few days.
- There are signs of dehydration, such as excessive thirst, dark urine, or dizziness.
- Diarrhea is accompanied by severe abdominal pain, fever, or bloody stools.

By combining these elements, you'll have a comprehensive approach to reclaiming digestive balance during episodes of diarrhea. "Health Is Wealth" remains dedicated to providing practical tools for your journey to a healthier, balanced life. In the subsequent chapters, we will explore additional facets of natural wellness, addressing various aspects of physical, mental, and emotional well-being.

It is crucial to stay hydrated during diarrhea and consume a combination of water, and electrolyte-rich fluids, and these natural remedies can contribute to symptom relief. If diarrhea persists or is severe, it's advisable to consult with a healthcare professional for proper evaluation and guidance.

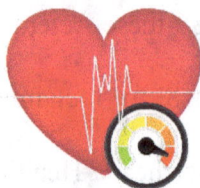

## Chapter 7: Natural Approaches to Managing Blood Pressure

In the symphony of health, the rhythm of our heart sets the tone for overall well-being. Chapter 7 of "Health Is Wealth" delves into the critical realm of blood pressure management, exploring natural approaches to empower your heart and promote cardiovascular health. Understanding the factors influencing blood pressure, embracing lifestyle modifications, and integrating specific herbs form the foundation of this comprehensive exploration.

Before we embark on the journey of natural approaches, let us grasp the significance of blood pressure as a vital indicator of cardiovascular health. Blood pressure measures the force exerted by blood against the walls of arteries, influencing the heart's workload.

Uncontrolled high blood pressure can lead to serious health complications such as hypertension, strokes, and heart attacks, underscoring the importance of proactive management. Here are a few lifestyle modifications that can help regulate blood pressure:

**1. Mindful Eating:**
Cultivating awareness around dietary choices is a cornerstone of heart health. Embrace a diet rich in whole foods, emphasizing fruits, vegetables, whole grains, and lean proteins. Adopting the DASH (Dietary Approaches to Stop Hypertension) principles can be particularly beneficial in managing blood pressure.

**2. Regular Physical Activity:**
Incorporate regular exercise into your routine to promote cardiovascular fitness. Activities such as brisk walking, swimming, or cycling can contribute to maintaining a healthy blood pressure range.

**3. Stress Management:**

Chronic stress can elevate blood pressure. Explore stress-reducing practices such as meditation, deep breathing exercises, and yoga to foster a calmer mental and emotional state.

**4. Maintaining a Healthy Weight:**

Achieving and maintaining a healthy weight is pivotal for blood pressure management. Focus on a balanced diet and regular exercise to support weight maintenance.

This chapter guides you in crafting a personalized toolkit for heart empowerment, encompassing lifestyle modifications, specific herbs, and proactive monitoring. By embracing these natural approaches, you embark on a journey to empower your heart and foster cardiovascular well-being. Here are a few herbs for blood pressure support:

**1. Hawthorn Berry:**

Hawthorn berry has a long history of use in traditional medicine for heart health.

It is believed to improve blood flow, strengthen the heart, and lower blood pressure. Incorporating hawthorn berries into your routine, either as a supplement or tea, can be a natural approach to support cardiovascular well-being.

### 2. Olive Leaf Extract:

Rich in antioxidants, olive leaf extract has been associated with potential benefits for blood pressure regulation. Consider incorporating olive leaf extract as a supplement, ensuring it aligns with your overall health plan.

### 3. Garlic:

Known for its cardiovascular benefits, garlic may help lower blood pressure and improve circulation. Raw garlic or garlic supplements can be considered as a flavorful addition to meals or as a supplement for cardiovascular support.

## 4. Beetroot:

Beetroot contains nitric oxide, which may help dilate blood vessels and improve blood flow, contributing to healthy blood pressure levels. Fresh beetroot juice or incorporating beets into your diet can be a delicious way to harness its potential benefits.

## 5. Fish Oil:

Omega-3 fatty acids present in fish oil may have a positive impact on blood pressure. Consider incorporating fatty fish such as salmon, mackerel, or taking fish oil supplements after consulting with healthcare professionals.

## 6. Celery Seed Extract:

Celery seed extract has been traditionally used to support cardiovascular health. Its potential diuretic effect may contribute to lower blood pressure. Consult with healthcare professionals before adding celery seed extract to your regimen.

**7. Oregano:**

Oregano contains compounds that may help relax blood vessels, potentially contributing to blood pressure regulation. Use fresh or dried oregano in your culinary creations for both flavor and potential health benefits.

**8. Hibiscus Tea:**

Research suggests that hibiscus tea may have antihypertensive properties, aiding in blood pressure reduction. Enjoying hibiscus tea as part of your daily hydration routine can be a refreshing way to support heart health.

**9. Cocoa:**

Dark chocolate and cocoa products contain flavonoids that may contribute to blood pressure regulation. Opt for high-quality dark chocolate with at least 70% cocoa content as an occasional treat.

Empowerment begins with awareness. Consider investing in a home blood pressure monitor to track your blood pressure regularly. This proactive approach enables you to observe trends, monitor the effectiveness of lifestyle modifications, and collaborate with healthcare professionals for optimal management.

While natural approaches can complement blood pressure management, it's essential to consult with healthcare professionals for personalized guidance. Discuss your health goals, share your natural approaches, and work collaboratively to achieve and maintain optimal blood pressure levels.

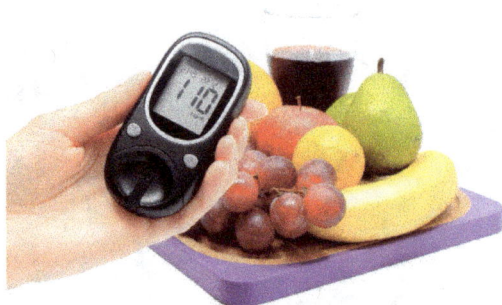

# Chapter 8: Diabetes Management: Balancing Blood Sugar

Navigating the complex landscape of diabetes requires a multifaceted approach that extends beyond conventional interventions. Chapter 8 of "Health Is Wealth" dives into the realm of balancing blood sugar with a holistic approach. Understanding the nuances of diabetes management, embracing lifestyle modifications, exploring specific herbs and fruits, and incorporating intermittent fasting create a comprehensive guide for those seeking holistic remedies to diabetes care.

Before delving into remedies and holistic approaches, let's unravel the complexity of diabetes.

Whether Type 1 or Type 2, diabetes involves the body's inability to regulate blood sugar effectively. Lifestyle factors, genetics, and environmental influences contribute to the onset and progression of diabetes. Here are the key lifestyle modifications for successful diabetes management:

**1. Balanced Diet:**

Adopting a balanced diet is foundational for managing blood sugar levels. Emphasize whole foods, lean proteins, high-fiber grains, and plenty of vegetables. Monitor carbohydrate intake and opt for complex carbohydrates to promote stable blood sugar.

**2. Regular Physical Activity:**

Exercise plays a pivotal role in diabetes management. Engage in regular physical activity to improve insulin sensitivity and help regulate blood sugar. Activities like walking, swimming, or yoga can be tailored to individual preferences and health conditions.

### 3. Stress Management:

Chronic stress can impact blood sugar levels. Incorporate stress-reducing practices such as meditation, deep breathing exercises, and mindfulness to create a calmer mental and emotional state.

### 4. Adequate Sleep:

Quality sleep is integral for overall health, including blood sugar regulation. Strive for 7-9 hours of uninterrupted sleep each night to support optimal well-being.

Each previously mentioned lifestyle modification is extremely crucial in the fight against diabetes, none of which should be taken lightly. Along with lifestyle modifications, these are a few herbs and fruits that help regulate Blood Sugar.

### 1. Cinnamon:

Cinnamon has shown potential in improving insulin sensitivity and lowering blood sugar levels.

Incorporate cinnamon into your diet, either by sprinkling it on foods or adding it to beverages.

### 2. Fenugreek:

Fenugreek seeds contain soluble fiber that may help lower blood sugar levels. Consider adding fenugreek to your diet or taking it as a supplement, following healthcare professional guidance.

### 3. Bitter Melon:

Bitter melon has been traditionally used to lower blood sugar levels. Whether consumed as a vegetable or in supplement form, bitter melon may offer support for diabetes management.

### 4. Berberine:

Derived from several plants, including goldenseal and barberry, berberine has demonstrated potential in regulating blood sugar levels. Consult with healthcare professionals before incorporating berberine into your regimen.

### 5. Turmeric:

Curcumin, the active compound in turmeric, exhibits anti-inflammatory and blood sugar-regulating properties. Consider incorporating turmeric into your cooking or taking it as a supplement after consulting with healthcare professionals.

### 6. Berries:

Berries, such as blueberries, strawberries, and raspberries, are rich in antioxidants and fiber. They contribute to stable blood sugar levels and can be enjoyed as a delicious snack or added to meals.

### 7. Apples:

Apples contain soluble fiber, which slows down the digestion and absorption of carbohydrates, aiding in blood sugar regulation. Enjoying a fresh apple as a snack or adding slices to your oatmeal can be a delightful way to include this fruit.

### 8. Avocado:

Avocado is a nutrient-dense fruit that provides healthy monounsaturated fats. Its low-carbohydrate content and high fiber make it a suitable choice for blood sugar management. Add avocado slices to salads or enjoy it as a spread.

Now that we have discussed fruits and herbs, let us now briefly discuss the valuable relationship between fasting and diabetes. For the sake of this chapter, we will focus on intermittent fasting. Intermittent fasting involves cycles of eating and fasting, potentially offering benefits for blood sugar control. However, individuals with diabetes, especially at higher levels or with complications, should approach fasting cautiously and under the guidance of healthcare professionals.

There are different types of intermittent fasting options to choose from. For example, there is time-restricted eating, which involves limiting daily eating to a specific time window, such as an 8-hour period which can support blood sugar regulation.

Alternate-day fasting, which involves alternating between days of regular eating and days with significantly reduced calorie intake, may provide extreme benefits for some individuals.

Next, there is what is called 5:2 fasting, which involves eating normally for five days and restricting calorie intake to a minimal level on two non-consecutive days. The benefits of intermittent fasting are as follows:

1. Improved insulin sensitivity.
2. Enhanced cellular repair and regeneration.
3. Regulation of hormones involved in blood sugar control.

### Here are 3 main Considerations for Fasting and Diabetes:

1. Monitor blood sugar levels regularly, especially during fasting periods.

2. Stay hydrated and ensure adequate nutrient intake during eating windows.
3. Collaborate with healthcare professionals to tailor fasting approaches to individual health needs.

This chapter guides you in crafting a personalized toolkit for holistic diabetes management, encompassing lifestyle modifications, specific herbs, fruits, and the potential exploration of intermittent fasting. Empower yourself with knowledge, collaborate with healthcare professionals, and embark on a holistic journey toward balancing blood sugar and promoting overall well-being.

"Health Is Wealth" remains dedicated to providing practical tools for your journey to a healthier, balanced life. In the upcoming chapters, we will continue to explore various facets of natural wellness, addressing physical, mental, and emotional well-being.

## Disclaimer

Before exploring intermittent fasting or making significant changes to your lifestyle, especially if diabetes is at a higher level or involves severe complications, it is imperative to consult with healthcare professionals. They can provide personalized guidance, monitor your progress, and ensure that any interventions align with your overall health plan.

## Chapter 9: Health Benefits of Vinegar and Apple Cider Vinegar

Chapter 9 of "Health Is Wealth" invites you to explore the tangy wonders of vinegar, particularly focusing on the acclaimed elixir, apple cider vinegar, also known as (ACV). From digestive support to potential blood sugar regulation, and weight loss, vinegar emerges as a versatile companion on your journey to holistic health and well-being.

### The Health Benefits of Vinegar:

### 1. Digestive Aid:

- Vinegar may enhance digestion by promoting the production of stomach acid, aiding in the breakdown of food.

**2. Blood Sugar Regulation:**

- Some studies suggest that vinegar, including ACV, may help regulate blood sugar levels, potentially beneficial for those with diabetes or insulin resistance.

**3. Weight Management:**

- Consuming vinegar with meals may contribute to increased feelings of fullness, potentially supporting weight management efforts.

**4. Heart Health:**

- ACV may have a positive impact on heart health by supporting cholesterol levels and blood pressure regulation.

**5. Antioxidant Boost:**

- The antioxidants in vinegar help combat oxidative stress, protecting cells from damage.

### 6. Immune Support:

- Vinegar's antimicrobial properties may contribute to immune system support, potentially aiding in the prevention of infections.

### Types of Vinegar and Their Benefits:

### 1. Apple Cider Vinegar (ACV):

- Digestive Tonic: Mix 1-2 tablespoons of ACV with water before meals to enhance digestion.
- Blood Sugar Support: Dilute 1-2 tablespoons of ACV in water and consume before meals for potential blood sugar regulation.

### 2. White Vinegar:

- Cleaning Agent: Mix with water as a natural and effective cleaning solution for surfaces.

### 3. Balsamic Vinegar:

- Salad Dressing: Use as a flavorful and antioxidant-rich base for salad dressings.

### 4. Red Wine Vinegar:

- Marinades: Create savory marinades for meats and vegetables.

### 5. Apple Cider Vinegar Capsules:

- ACV capsules offer a convenient option for those who find the liquid form unpalatable.

### Benefits of ACV Capsules:
### 1. Digestive Support:

- Take ACV capsules before meals to potentially enhance digestion and support nutrient absorption.

### 2. Blood Sugar Management:

- Capsules can provide the benefits of ACV for blood sugar regulation without the taste.

**3. Weight Management:**

- Consistent use of ACV capsules may contribute to feelings of fullness, supporting weight management goals.

### How to Incorporate Vinegar into Your Routine

**1. Morning Elixir:**

- Start your day with a warm cup of water, a tablespoon of ACV, and a drizzle of honey for a refreshing morning elixir.

**2. Salad Dressings:**

- Create delicious and nutritious salad dressings using different types of vinegar for added flavor.

**3. Marinades and Sauces:**

- Enhance the taste of your favorite dishes by incorporating vinegar into marinades and sauces.

### 4. Capsule Routine:

- If the taste of ACV is not appealing, consider integrating ACV capsules into your daily supplement routine.

This chapter guides you in crafting a personalized wellness routine that embraces the health benefits of vinegar and ACV. Explore the versatility of this tangy elixir, whether in liquid or capsule form and savor the many ways it can enhance your journey to holistic well-being.

"Health Is Wealth" continues to unfold as a comprehensive guide, offering insights and practical tools for your journey to a healthier, more balanced life. Here are 2 main things to remember when consuming vinegar or ACV:

### 1. Moderation:

- While vinegar offers numerous benefits, excessive consumption may have adverse effects. Use in moderation.

## 2. <u>Dilution</u>:

- Always dilute vinegar, especially ACV, when consuming it in liquid form to protect tooth enamel and the esophagus.

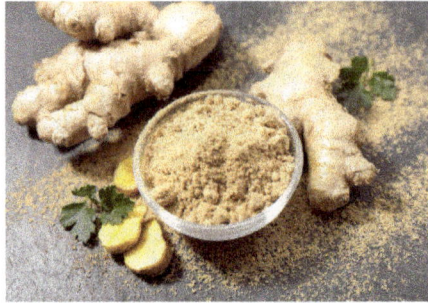

## ***Chapter 10: Health Benefits of Ginger***

Welcome to Chapter 10 of "Health Is Wealth," where we dive into the zesty world of ginger. Whether in its whole natural form, powdered, minced, or encapsulated form, ginger unveils a plethora of health benefits, adding not just flavor but a burst of wellness to your daily life.

In its whole, unadulterated form, ginger is a root that has been revered for centuries across cultures for its distinctive taste and remarkable health properties. Let's explore the vibrant benefits it brings to the table:

**1. Digestive Dynamo:**

- Ginger stimulates the production of digestive juices, aiding in the breakdown of food and alleviating indigestion.

**2. Anti-Inflammatory Warrior:**

- Rich in gingerol, a bioactive compound, ginger exhibits potent anti-inflammatory properties, potentially reducing inflammation in the body.

**3. Nausea Soother:**

- Whether from motion sickness, morning sickness, or general nausea, ginger can be a natural remedy to soothe unsettled stomachs.

**4. Immune Booster:**

- Packed with antioxidants, ginger supports the immune system, helping the body fend off infections.

**5. Pain Relief Partner:**

- The anti-inflammatory properties extend to pain relief, making ginger a natural ally for managing various types of pain.

**Powdered and Minced Ginger:**

In its powdered or minced forms, ginger unveils its culinary versatility while retaining its health benefits:

**1. Cooking Companion:**

- Sprinkle powdered ginger into your dishes for a burst of flavor and potential health perks.

**2. Tea Time Treat:**

- Create a soothing cup of ginger tea by infusing powdered or minced ginger in hot water, promoting relaxation and digestion.

### 3. Flavorful Spice Blend:

- Blend minced ginger into spice mixes to enhance the taste of your favorite recipes, from savory dishes to desserts.

### 4. Baking Brilliance:

- Incorporate powdered ginger into baking recipes, infusing your treats with warmth and potential health benefits.

### Ginger in Capsule Form:

For those seeking the benefits of ginger without the strong taste, encapsulated ginger provides a convenient solution:

### 1. Digestive Support:

- Ginger capsules offer a simple way to support digestion, especially for those who find the taste too intense.

### 2. Travel Companion:

- Take ginger capsules while traveling to help alleviate motion sickness or nausea.

### 3. Daily Wellness Boost:

- Integrate ginger capsules into your daily supplement routine for consistent support to your overall well-being.

### 4. Anti-Inflammatory Aid:

- Capsules can provide a concentrated dose of ginger's anti-inflammatory properties for those managing inflammation.

### Conversational Insights:

Now that we've journeyed through the diverse forms of ginger, let's appreciate its charm and practicality. Imagine adding a touch of freshly minced ginger to your soup, sipping on a steaming cup of ginger tea, or simply popping a ginger capsule to kickstart your day.

Picture yourself peeling a piece of fresh ginger, feeling the aroma awaken your senses. The root's knobby exterior hides a burst of flavor and wellness waiting to be unleashed in your culinary creations.

Consider the convenience of a jar of powdered ginger or a packet of minced ginger, ready to sprinkle onto your meals. The kitchen transforms into a haven of aromatic delights, and your taste buds dance with each bite. For those days when the strong taste of ginger doesn't quite align with your palate, imagine the simplicity of reaching for a jar of ginger capsules. Pop one with a glass of water, and you're set for a day filled with ginger's potential benefits.

Whether you're drawn to the whole natural form, the convenience of powdered or minced ginger, or the simplicity of capsules, ginger invites you to infuse your life with its zesty charm.

Experiment with recipes, brew a comforting cup of ginger tea or seamlessly incorporate ginger capsules into your daily routine.

## *Chapter 11: The Multifaceted Benefits of Turmeric*

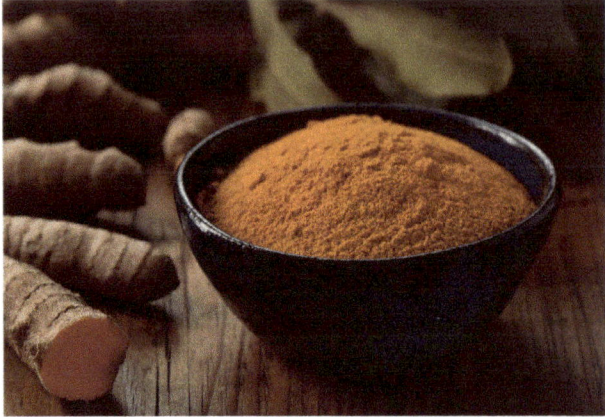

Welcome to Chapter 11 of "Health Is Wealth," where we explore the radiant world of turmeric—a golden elixir celebrated for its versatile health benefits. From its anti-inflammatory prowess to its potential role in mental well-being, turmeric takes center stage as a holistic wellness companion. The health benefits of turmeric are as follows:

### 1. Anti-Inflammatory Powerhouse:

- Curcumin, the active compound in turmeric, exhibits potent anti-inflammatory properties, potentially reducing inflammation and its associated risks.
### 2. Antioxidant Defender:

- Turmeric is rich in antioxidants, combating oxidative stress and protecting cells from damage.

**3. Joint Support:**

- The anti-inflammatory nature of turmeric may contribute to joint health, potentially alleviating symptoms of arthritis.

**4. Heart Health Ally:**

- Turmeric may support heart health by improving blood vessel function and regulating cholesterol levels.

**5. Brain Boost:**

- Curcumin's neuroprotective properties may enhance cognitive function and reduce the risk of neurodegenerative diseases.

**6. Digestive Harmony:**

- Turmeric promotes digestive health by stimulating bile production and aiding in the breakdown of fats.

### 7. <u>Balancing Blood Sugar</u>:

- Preliminary studies suggest that turmeric may assist in balancing blood sugar levels, offering potential benefits for those with diabetes.

### 8. <u>Skin Radiance</u>:

- Turmeric's anti-inflammatory and antioxidant properties may contribute to healthy and radiant skin.

### 9. <u>Mood Support</u>:

- Some research indicates that curcumin may have antidepressant effects, potentially supporting mental well-being.

### <u>Varieties of Turmeric and Their Unique Qualities</u>:

### 1. <u>Raw Turmeric Root</u>:

- Peel and grate raw turmeric to add to smoothies or salads for a fresh and vibrant boost.

### 2. <u>Turmeric Powder</u>:

- A versatile option for cooking, turmeric powder adds color and flavor to various dishes, from curries to soups.

### 3. <u>Turmeric Capsules</u>:

- Capsules offer a convenient way to incorporate turmeric into your daily supplement routine, ensuring consistent intake.
  **4. Turmeric Tea:**

- Steep grated or powdered turmeric in hot water for a soothing and aromatic cup of turmeric tea.
  **5. Turmeric Extract:**

- Extracts concentrate curcumin, providing a potent form for those seeking higher concentrations of this beneficial compound.

**Recipes to Savor Turmeric's Goodness:**

**1. Golden Turmeric Latte:**

- **Ingredients:**
  1 cup almond or coconut milk
  1 teaspoon turmeric powder
  1/2 teaspoon cinnamon
  A pinch of black pepper
  1 teaspoon honey or maple syrup (optional)
- **Instructions:**
  Heat the milk in a saucepan.Whisk in turmeric, cinnamon, and black pepper. Simmer for a few minutes, then sweeten to taste.

## 2. Turmeric-Spiced Quinoa Bowl:

- **Ingredients:**
  1 cup cooked quinoa
  1/2 cup roasted vegetables (e.g., sweet potatoes, broccoli)
  1/4 cup chickpeas, cooked
  1 teaspoon turmeric powder
  Olive oil, salt, and pepper to taste
- **Instructions:**
  Toss cooked quinoa, roasted vegetables, and chickpeas in a bowl. Drizzle with olive oil and sprinkle turmeric powder, salt, and pepper. Mix well and enjoy a nutritious turmeric-spiced bowl.

### 3. Turmeric and Ginger Infused Water:

- **Ingredients:**
  1 teaspoon grated turmeric
  1 teaspoon grated ginger
  Slices of lemon
  Mint leaves
  Water and ice
- **Instructions:**
  Combine grated turmeric and ginger in a jug. Add lemon slices, mint leaves, and ice. Fill with water, stir, and let it infuse for refreshing hydration.

### Crafting Your Turmeric Infusion

Whether you're sprinkling turmeric into your cooking, sipping on a golden latte, or incorporating capsules into your routine, turmeric invites you to infuse your life with its radiant charm. Embrace its culinary and wellness versatility, and let the golden elixir weave its magic.

## Chapter 12: The Sweet Benefits of Cinnamon

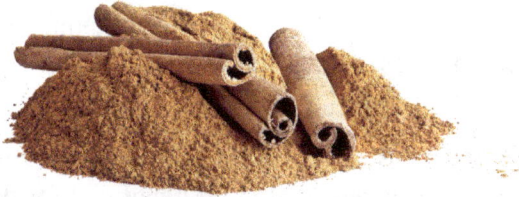

Welcome to Chapter 12 of "Health Is Wealth," where we will explore the sweet and aromatic world of cinnamon—a spice not just world-renowned for its culinary allure, but also celebrated for its diverse health benefits and remedies. Let's dive into the warm embrace of cinnamon and discover how it can enrich your journey to holistic well-being.

### The Bountiful Health Benefits of Cinnamon:

### 1. Antioxidant Abundance:

- Cinnamon is rich in antioxidants that combat oxidative stress, protecting cells from damage.

**2. Anti-Inflammatory Marvel:**

- The anti-inflammatory properties of cinnamon may help reduce inflammation in the body.

**3. Blood Sugar Regulation:**

- Cinnamon has shown promise in helping regulate blood sugar levels, making it beneficial for those with diabetes or insulin resistance.

**4. Heart Health Support:**

- Cinnamon may contribute to heart health by improving cholesterol levels and reducing the risk of heart disease.

**5. Cognitive Boost:**

- Preliminary research suggests that cinnamon may enhance cognitive function and memory.

**6. Anti-Microbial Magic:**

- Cinnamon possesses antimicrobial properties, potentially aiding in the prevention of infections.

**7. Digestive Comfort:**

- Cinnamon may help alleviate digestive discomfort by reducing bloating and aiding in digestion.

**8. Joint Wellness:**

- The anti-inflammatory nature of cinnamon may provide relief for joint pain and inflammation.

**Remedies and Practical Uses of Cinnamon:**

**1. Cinnamon Tea for Digestive Ease:**

- Brew a cup of cinnamon tea by steeping a cinnamon stick or a teaspoon of ground cinnamon in hot water. Enjoy before or after meals for digestive comfort.

## 2. Blood Sugar-Balancing Smoothie:

- Create a nutritious smoothie by blending Greek yogurt, berries, a banana, and a sprinkle of cinnamon. This delightful blend may contribute to blood sugar regulation.

## 3. Anti-Inflammatory Golden Milk:

- Prepare a soothing golden milk by combining coconut milk, turmeric, a dash of cinnamon, and a hint of honey. Sip on this comforting elixir to harness the anti-inflammatory benefits of cinnamon.

## 4. Cinnamon-infused Honey for Immunity:

- Infuse honey with cinnamon by mixing a teaspoon of ground cinnamon into a jar of honey. Allow it to sit for a few days. Use this cinnamon-infused honey as a sweet and immune-boosting addition to your beverages or drizzled on toast.

## 5. Joint Massage Oil:

- Create a joint-friendly massage oil by mixing a few drops of cinnamon essential oil with a carrier oil, such as coconut or almond oil. Massage this blend onto joints for potential relief from inflammation.

**6. <u>Cinnamon and Honey Face Mask</u>:**

- Mix ground cinnamon with honey to create a natural face mask. Apply it to your face, let it sit for 15-20 minutes, and rinse off. This mask may promote skin health and a radiant complexion.

**<u>Embracing Cinnamon's Versatility</u>:**

Cinnamon, with its warm and inviting aroma, brings not only a delightful taste to food and beverages but also a host of wellness benefits. Picture the comforting sight of a steaming cup of cinnamon tea or the delectable aroma of cinnamon-infused honey. Let's savor the sweet essence of cinnamon as it weaves its therapeutic magic into our lives.

Whether you're indulging in a cup of tea, concocting a blood sugar-balancing smoothie, or pampering your skin with a cinnamon and honey face mask, cinnamon invites you to infuse your routine with its warmth and goodness.

Embrace its versatility, and let the sweet essence of cinnamon enhance your journey to holistic well-being.

## <u>Chapter 13: Natural Antibiotics</u>

Step into Chapter 13 of "Health Is Wealth," where we unveil the natural arsenal of antibiotics bestowed upon us by the creator of earth and heaven! From the pungent power of garlic to the layers of goodness in onions, explore the diverse and potent benefits of these culinary gems that not only enhance flavor but also fortify your health.

### <u>Garlic: A Potent Natural Antibiotic</u>

**1. <u>Allicin Marvel</u>:**

Garlic contains allicin, a powerful compound known for its antibacterial, antiviral, and antifungal properties.

**2. Immune Support:**

- The allicin in garlic supports immune function, helping the body fend off infections.

**3. Cardiovascular Guardian:**

- Garlic may contribute to heart health by improving cholesterol levels and supporting blood vessel function.

**4. Anti-Inflammatory Ally:**

- Garlic exhibits anti-inflammatory effects, potentially aiding in the reduction of inflammation in the body.

**5. Digestive Harmony:**

- Consuming garlic may promote digestive health by supporting the balance of gut bacteria.

### Onions: Layers of Antibacterial Goodness

**1. Quercetin Boost:**

- Onions are rich in quercetin, an antioxidant with antibacterial and anti-inflammatory properties.

**2. Respiratory Wellness:**

- Quercetin in onions may support respiratory health, making them beneficial for conditions like allergies and asthma.

**3. Heart Health Guardian:**

- Onions contribute to heart health by potentially reducing cholesterol levels and supporting blood vessel function.

**4. Anti-Infection Properties:**

- The antibacterial properties of onions make them a natural ally in preventing and combating infections.

### The Heavenly Antibiotic Ensemble

**1. Honey:**

- Raw honey exhibits antibacterial properties and can be applied topically for wound healing.

### 2. Ginger:

- Ginger's antimicrobial properties make it a natural antibiotic, potentially aiding in the prevention of infections.

### 3. Turmeric:

- Curcumin in turmeric offers antibacterial and anti-inflammatory benefits, supporting overall health.

### 4. Oregano:

- Oregano contains compounds like carvacrol with antibacterial properties, making it a potent natural antibiotic.

### 5. Echinacea:

- Echinacea is known for its immune-boosting properties, helping the body resist infections.

## The Antibiotic Symphony:

Imagine the buttery flavor of fresh garlic bread made from scratch, or the savory aroma of onions in a sauté pan. These everyday ingredients not only add zest to your recipes but also orchestrate a symphony of health benefits. Let's explore the delightful and healing ensemble of nature's antibiotics.

Whether you're savoring a garlic-infused meal, adding the piquancy of onions to your dishes, or incorporating other natural antibiotics like honey, ginger, turmeric, oregano, and echinacea, nature invites you to infuse your life with its protective embrace. Embrace the flavors and benefits of these culinary gems, and let nature's antibiotics fortify your journey to holistic well-being.

# *Chapter 14: Embracing Holistic Habits for Optimal Health*

As we step into the final chapter of "Health Is Wealth," we unravel the profound advantages of embracing holistic habits for a healthier, more fulfilling, and balanced life. Beyond the conventional approaches, holistic living extends an invitation to nurture not just the body, but the mind and spirit as well.

## The Foundations of Holistic Habits:

### 1. Mind-Body Harmony:

- Holistic habits recognize the intricate dance between the mind and body, acknowledging that mental well-being profoundly influences physical health.

## 2. Prevention as a Priority:

- Rather than solely addressing symptoms, holistic habits prioritize preventing imbalances and ailments, fostering a proactive approach to health.

## 3. Individualized Wellness:

- Holistic living appreciates the uniqueness of each individual, recognizing that what works for one may not work for another. It encourages personalized approaches to well-being.

## 4. Nutrient-Dense Nutrition:

- Holistic habits emphasize nourishing the body with whole, nutrient-dense foods, providing the essential building blocks for optimal health.

**5. Physical Activity with Purpose:**

- Exercise in holistic living goes beyond mere physical activity; it becomes a mindful practice that aligns with individual needs, promoting strength, flexibility, and overall vitality.

**6. Stress Management Strategies:**

- Holistic habits address stress as a multifaceted challenge, incorporating diverse strategies such as mindfulness, meditation, and relaxation techniques.

**The Holistic Advantage:**

**1. Balanced Energy Flow:**

- Practices like acupuncture, yoga, and energy healing in holistic living aim to balance the body's energy flow, promoting overall well-being.

**2. Emotional Resilience:**

- Holistic habits nurture emotional resilience, fostering the ability to navigate life's challenges with grace and balance.

**3. Connection to Nature:**

- Recognizing the profound connection between humans and nature, holistic living encourages spending time outdoors, grounding practices, and fostering a deeper appreciation for the natural world.

**4. Spiritual Fulfillment:**

- Whether through religious practices, meditation, or mindful rituals, holistic habits provide avenues for spiritual exploration and fulfillment.

**5. Community and Social Well-Being:**

- Holistic living acknowledges the impact of social connections on health, fostering a sense of community and supportive relationships.

**Chapter Conclusion:**

Whether you're embracing mindful eating, incorporating holistic therapies, or cultivating emotional resilience, holistic living invites you to compose your own unique symphony of well-being. Hopefully, the chapters of

"Health Is Wealth" have guided you through the realms of natural remedies, nutritional wisdom, and holistic practices, providing a comprehensive guide to a life infused with vitality.

"Health Is Wealth" unfolds as a testament to the profound wisdom and richness that holistic living offers. In the chapters you've explored, you've witnessed the fusion of ancient practices, modern insights, and the timeless wisdom of God and Mother Nature. May your path be illuminated by the radiance of the sun, guiding you toward a life of optimal health, wealth, and prosperity.

## *Final Thoughts*

Holistic health is not a new concept; it's an ancient wisdom that recognizes the intricate connection between our mental, physical, and spiritual well-being. Understanding this symbiotic relationship lays the foundation for the transformative journey that awaits you. We have navigated the fundamental principles of natural healing, emphasizing the importance of balance and harmony. Nature, with its myriad herbs and substances, becomes our ally in achieving and maintaining this equilibrium.

As you reflect on the wisdom shared within these chapters, may you find inspiration to embrace the simplicity and richness that holistic living offers.

It's a journey where the nourishment of mind, body, and spirit converges, and where the profound symphony of natural remedies and holistic practices orchestrates a life of vitality, balance, and joy. Please remember the significance of embracing a lifestyle that aligns with the rhythms of the natural world, a lifestyle that is not just about treating symptoms, but fostering overall well-being, as well as preventative measures.

No one should have to take medication with harmful side-effects for the remainder of their lives! "Health Is Wealth" is dedicated to helping people take control of their destiny. If you enjoyed the content of this book, please take the time to give it a review on Amazon or whatever platform you got it from. I thank you for taking this journey with me.

May your path be illuminated by the glow of holistic living, guiding you toward a life where each day becomes an inspirational chapter in the story of your well-being. As you step forward, may you carry the transformative insights and nurturing wisdom of "Health Is Wealth" with you as you travel through your holistic journey.

With gratitude for your presence on this odyssey of well-being,

*Charles Lovjoy*

Author, "Health Is Wealth: Holistic Home Remedies."

# *Other Works:*

## Paperback, Hard-cover, e-books, and audiobooks

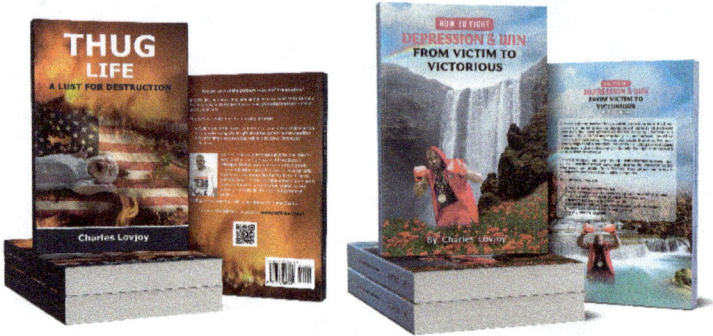

## *Introducing MG KIDS coloring books*

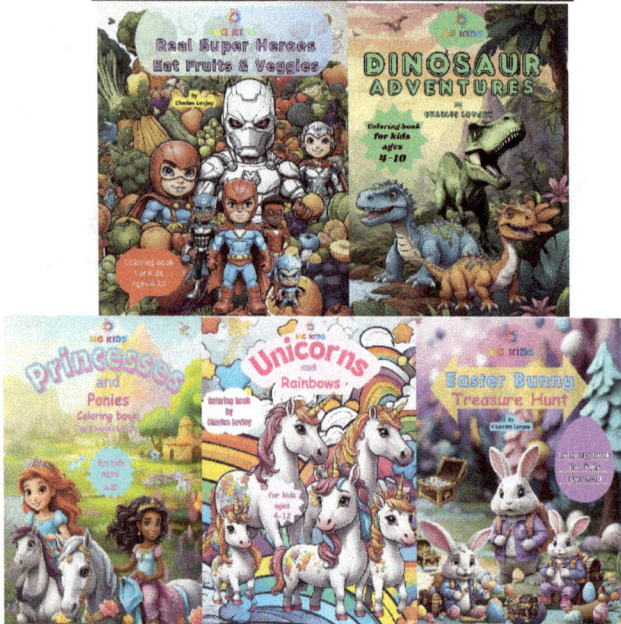

## <u>Music available on all digital platforms</u>!

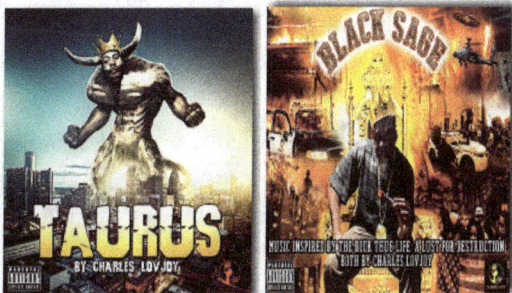

### Movies & TV shows

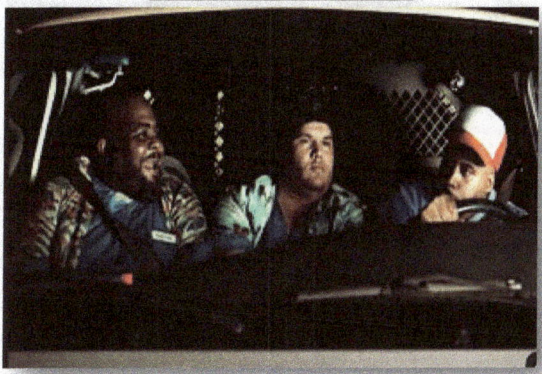

Watch Charles Lovjoy in the hit comedy series "Detroiters," Season 1–episode #9 "THE GREAT ESCAPE." Available on PARAMOUNT PLUS. Originally aired on the COMEDY CENTRAL NETWORK

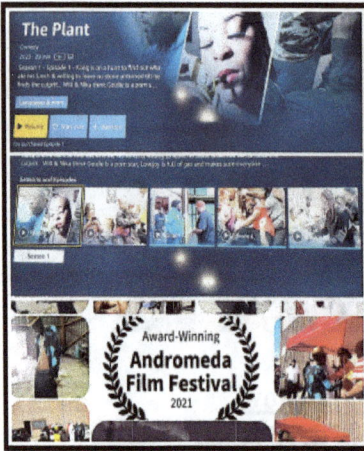

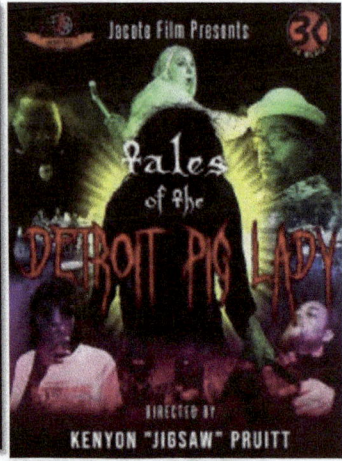

Also watch Charles Lovjoy in these shows available on:

- Amazon Prime Video

- Tubi TV

- Pluto TV

- The Roku Channel

## *References and Citations*

**Books**:

Foster, R., & Johnson, D. V. (2006). "Desk Reference to Nature's Medicine." National Geographic Society.

The staff of FC&A (2008). The Cure Conspiracy" FC&A Publishing.

Murray, M. T., & Pizzorno, J. E. (2012). "The Encyclopedia of Natural Medicine." Atria Books.

Charles Lovjoy (2022). "How To Fight Depression and Win: From Victim To Victorious." Muscle Gang Publications.

## Journal Articles:

Haniadka, R., Saldanha, E., Sunita, V., Palatty, P. L., Fayad, R., & Baliga, M. S. (2013). A review of the gastroprotective effects of ginger (Zingiber officinale Roscoe). **Food & Function, 4(6), 845-855.**

Kiecolt-Glaser, J. K., Bennett, J. M., Andridge, R., Peng, J., Shapiro, C. L., Malarkey, W. B., & Emery, C. F. (2014). Yoga's impact on inflammation, mood, and fatigue in breast cancer survivors: a randomized controlled trial. Journal of Clinical Oncology, 32(10), 1040-1049.

## Scientific Papers:

Ali, B. H., Blunden, G., Tanira, M. O., & Nemmar, A. (2008). Some phytochemical, pharmacological and toxicological properties of ginger (Zingiber officinale Roscoe): a review of recent research. Food and Chemical Toxicology, 46(2), 409-420.

Ritchie, M. R., & Cummings, J. H. (2013). Role of the gut microbiota in health and chronic gastrointestinal disease: understanding a hidden metabolic organ. Therapeutic Advances in Gastroenterology, 6(4), 295-308.

## Online Resources:

National Center for Complementary and Integrative Health. "Ginger." [https://www.nccih.nih.gov/health/ginger]

Mayo Clinic. "Diarrhea: Causes and Remedies." [https://www.mayoclinic.org/symptoms/diarrhea/basics/causes/sym-20050926]

Healthline. "Home Remedies for Heartburn: What Works?" [https://www.healthline.com/health/gerd/home-remedies-for-heartburn]

World Health Organization. "Guidelines for Holistic Well-being." [https://www.who.int/health-topics]

CNBC "Sea moss health benefits" (2023) https://www.cnbc.com/2023/06/23/sea-moss-health-benefits-heres-what-the-science-says.html#:~:text=Other%20potential%20health%20benefits%20of,helps%20regulate%20your%20thyroid%20function.

Healthline (2023) https://www.healthline.com/nutrition/6-proven-health-benefits-of-apple-cider-vinegar

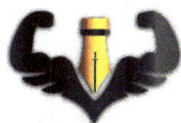

**MUSCLE GANG PUBLICATIONS**

*Charles Lovjoy*

www.ingramcontent.com/pod-product-compliance
Lightning Source LLC
Chambersburg PA
CBHW060907280326
41934CB00007B/1223